Lose weight by sleeping...

Following only 2 rules

It all started when a saleswoman at Manor in Vevey suggested a foolproof method to lose weight naturally so that I could then put on the undersized shirt I was trying to bring back to the store.

This method allowed her and her husband to lose weight in a few weeks, she assured me.

I was then able to test this method which made me lose 8 pounds in 4 weeks (about 0.4 pound / day) and allowed a very close friend to lose 37 pounds in 5 months.

The method is very easy to remember because it has only 2 rules that I will explain here in detail. The most complicated part is sometimes to put these 2 rules into practice, so this little manual should help you stay motivated throughout the process This little manual should help you stay motivated throughout the process of getting back to your teenage weight.

Enjoy your reading!

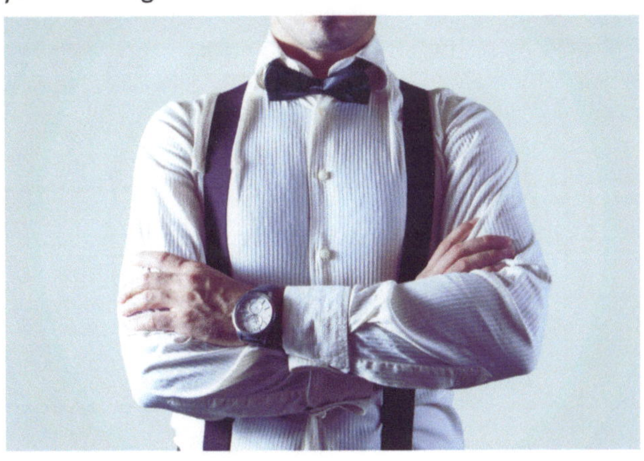

Contents

Chapter 1: The 2 Rules — **3**

Rule n°1 — 3

Rule n°2 — 4

Chapter 2: Preparation — **5**

Bullets to last — 6

An accurate Scale — 7

A regular measure — 8

A progression table — 9

Chapter 3: Boost your performance — **10**

Prioritize Some Vegetables — 11

A little exercise — 12

Final tip and conclusion — **13**

Appendixes — **14**

Starch list (to be excluded from 5:00 pm) — 14

Examples of Starch-Free Dishes — 15

Shopping list for 1 week — 16

Complete table to start well… — 17

Chapter 1
The 2 rules

Rule n°1

The first rule is the most important, it consists in **not eating starchy foods after 5:00 pm from Monday to Friday**. (By starchy foods, we mean legumes, cereals and tubers, so bread, pasta, rice, potatoes, etc.)*

The saleswoman told me that being Italian, she was used to eat pasta every night. She had to stop this habit in order to make it.

I was also used to have bread and cheese every night, and I can say that it's not so easy to avoid something as basic as bread.

To achieve this, a careful organization is necessary, it's all about knowing how to replace the element that we miss with something else...

But think about it, without starchy foods, you still have a lot of things to eat : vegetables, salads, meats, dairy products, eggs, etc.., there are still many choices!

The following pages will help you find your strategy for sticking to this rule until you reach your goal!

---

*For a more complete list, please see the appendixes.

Rule n°2

The second rule is simply **not to drink any sweetened beverage from Monday to Friday**.

In fact, a study conducted by various universities and hospitals in Switzerland (UNIGE, EPFL, HUG and CHUV)* recently revealed the correlation between the consumption of sweetened beverages and the risk of obesity*.

According to Albert Einstein, "success always comes when opportunity meets preparation". These 2 rules are a great opportunity to lose weight, so let's focus on preparation, the future key to your success!

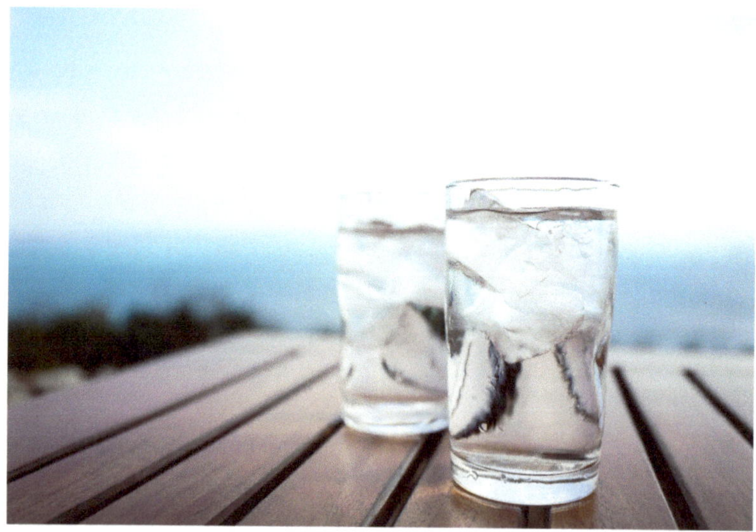

*https://www.unige.ch/communication/communiques/2019/quartiers-consommation-de-boissons-sucrees-et-obesite-lies/ (04.03.2022)

Chapter 2
The preparation

When you start a new method, there may be some small practical difficulties that can cause you to give up sooner than expected.

So let me share with you some very simple strategies to quickly put aside all these little obstacles.

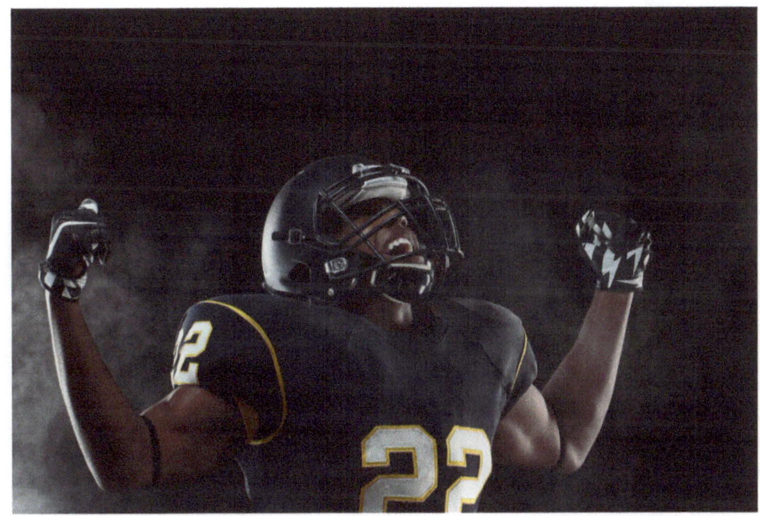

Bullets to Last

"You can't win a battle... without bullets", said Napoleon. To win this one, you must first arm yourself accordingly. The goal is not to go to bed hungry!

Before you go shopping, plan a menu of 5 meals without starches that you would like to eat on the evenings of this week. You will find some examples in the appendix of this leaflet. Once the plan is done, make a note of the quantities needed to prepare these meals and buy them at the beginning of your week so that you are ready for the battle!

Remember to keep it simple, especially if you are planning starchy meals for the rest of the family. You probably won't have the energy to make 2 different meals at the end of your day. To be sure you can do it, keep it simple and even prepare everything in advance. One last tip to keep you motivated: buy fresh, quality produce and wash it yourself. It takes more time, but it's so much better! And since it's all you're going to eat, the better it is, the more you will enjoy it ;-)

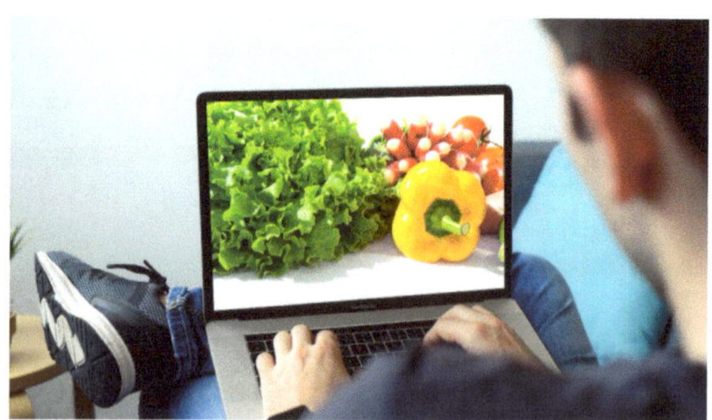

An Accurate Scale

The second thing to get is an accurate scale, capable of weighing you to within 0.1 lb. The easiest way to do this is to buy a digital scale that is usually available at low cost in the major retail stores. The problem with scales that only show pounds is that you will not be able to see your progress day by day, which will greatly help you stay motivated, especially in the beginning. In fact, the normal progression of this method represents a weight loss of 0.4 lb per day, and up to 2 lb in 5 days!

The most motivating thing is to be able to observe your daily progress in a tangible way, which is why having a scale that indicates your weight to within 0.1 lb is so important.

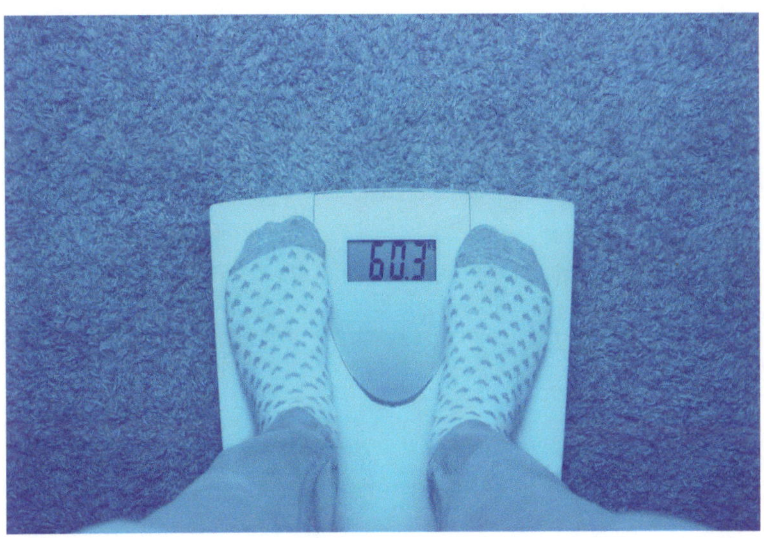

A Regular Measure

In order to measure your progress, you should also plan a time to take the measurement that is always the same. For example, in the morning, before showering, in your underwear, after going to the toilet. Your weight can easily vary by 0.4 lb if one of these parameters is not the same each time.

Keeping a regular time to weigh yourself will allow you to be absolutely sure of your progress day after day.

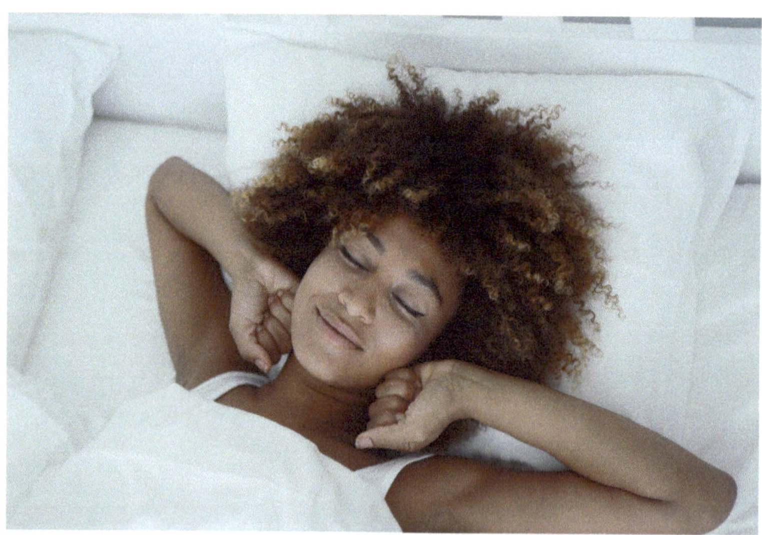

A progression table

In order to be able to visually see your progress and stay motivated throughout the journey, it is very important to be able to keep track of everything.

One of the possible methods is to draw a chart like this one in order to keep track of your weight progress every day. You will find several charts to complete in the appendixes.

Week	Mon	Tue	Wed	Thu	Fri	Sat	Sun
1	173.8	173.6	173.4	173.2	173.0		
2	172.8	172.6	172.4	172.2	172.0		
3	171.8	171.6	171.4	171.2	171.0		
4	170.8	170.6	170.4	170.2	170.0		

If you don't have the chart at hand when you weigh yourself, you can also simply dial the 3 digits above on your phone and start the call, your weight progress will then appear in your call history ;-)

Chapter 3
Boost your performance

With these 2 rules alone you should start to see results already after the 2nd week. But if you still have courage, you can of course accelerate the process. Here are a few simple suggestions that will help you significantly increase your progress.

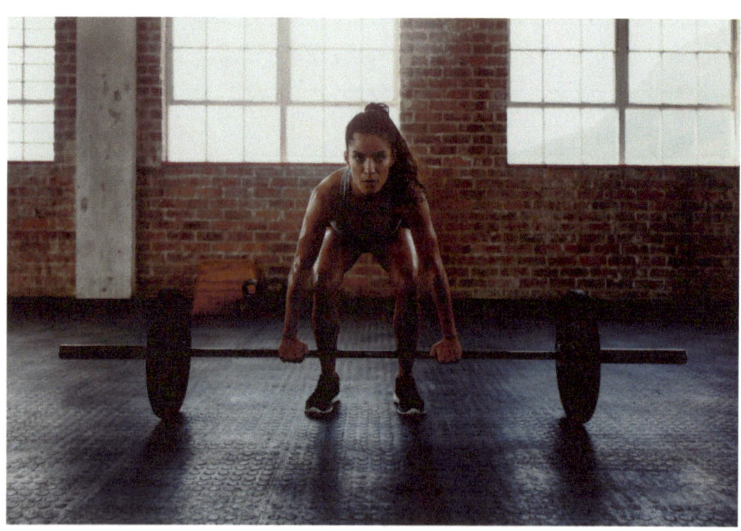

Focus on Certain Vegetables

With the experience we have found that some vegetables allow a better progression. It is about focusing on leafy vegetables (cabbage, spinach, lettuce, endive) and fruit vegetables (cucumber, eggplant, zucchini, tomato) which are naturally less dense in their structure and are therefore digested even more easily during the night.

If you want to get into high gear, you can therefore prioritize tomato or lettuce salads, rather than carrot or celery salads, but this is not an absolute rule, it is just a suggestion if you need a little "boost"!

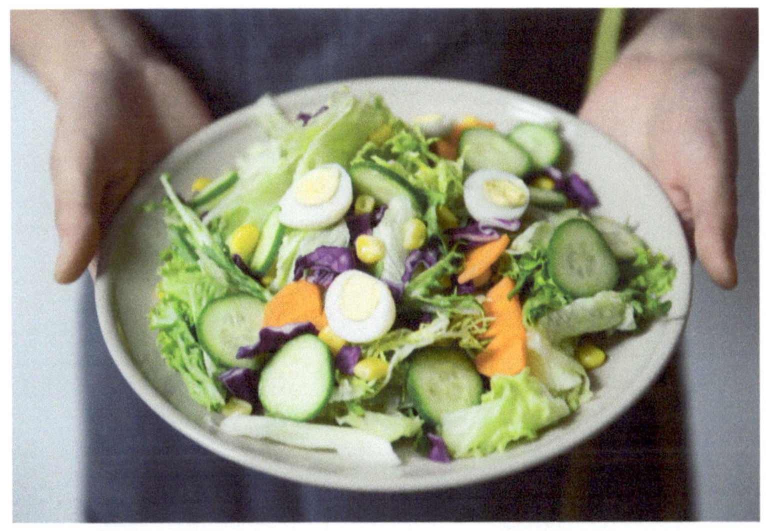

A little exercise

Our expertise also revealed that adding just 10 minutes of cardio (jogging, biking, etc...) per day could make you melt even faster. The 2 basic rules remain the same, these 10 minutes of endurance will only multiply the effect. This option can be very suitable for you if you start to find the time long :)

If you are not used to move at all, our advice is to use the SPE method (smallest possible effort). If 1 minute of jogging or biking makes you breathless, leave it at that level. Do it again the next day and only add a minute to the counter when the first one seems to easy. This will ensure you a natural progression towards your goal.

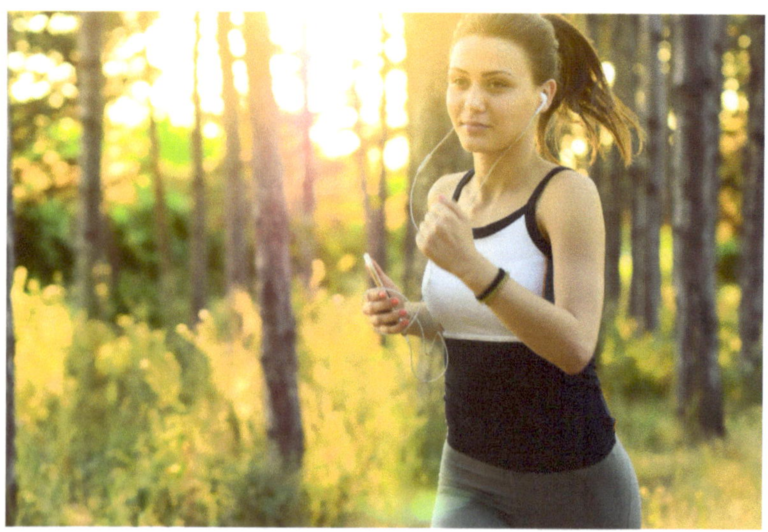

Final tips and conclusion

The principle of this method is simple, during the night, the body continues its digestion, but as the enzymes responsible for the digestion of starchy foods are mainly produced in the morning, your body will not digest starchy foods well during the night. When you stop eating starchy foods at night, digestion proceeds normally and you are left without the extra weight you used to store day after day. This also explains why weight loss stops when your accumulated fat is gone. So don't worry if you don't lose weight at all after a while, it's just that you have reached your ideal weight! Finally, note that the method also limits the production of insulin and therefore prevents diabetes and reduces the risk of cardiovascular disease.

It is now time to leave you and wish you a good start, the few appendixes that you will find here will help you to get started.

Lots of courage and above all plenty of fun!

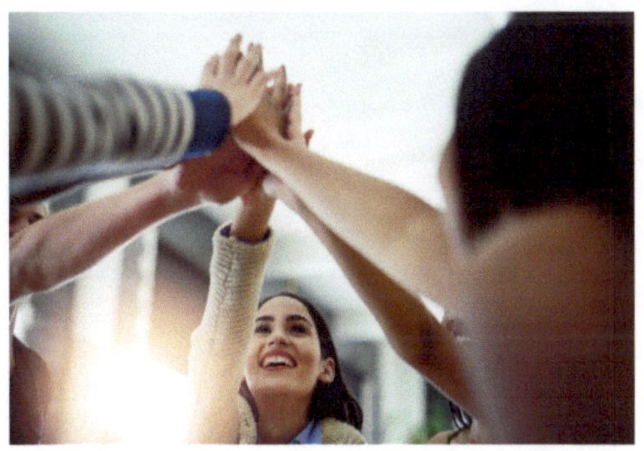

Appendixes

List of starches (to be excluded from 5:00 pm)

- Oats
- Wheat
- Spelt
- Broad beans
- Flageolets
- Beans
- Red, white and black beans
- Yam
- Lentils (green, coral...)
- Corn
- Cassava
- Millet
- Barley
- Sweet potato
- Chickpeas
- Yellow or green peas
- Potato
- Rice

Examples of Starch-Free Dishes

Caesar salad (lettuce, hard-boiled egg, parmesan cheese, chicken breast and Caesar sauce)

Niçoise salad (tomatoes, green peppers, garlic, onions, celery, artichoke, hard-boiled egg, anchovy fillets or tuna, black olives and olive oil or vinaigrette sauce)

Caprese salad (tomatoes, mozzarella, basil, olive oil or dressing)

Greek Salad (tomatoes, cucumber, oregano, feta, olives, onion, green bell pepper, capers, olive oil or dressing)

Mixed Salad (different kinds of lettuce, grated carrots, tomatoes, grated celery, feta or gruyere cheese, vinaigrette sauce)

Endive Salad (Endive, Gruyere cheese, raisins, apple pieces, tomatoes, vinaigrette)

Vinaigrette Sauce (⅔ extra virgin olive oil, ⅓ balsamic vinegar, 1 pinch of herbal salt, 1 pinch of herbes de Provence, 1 pinch of pepper, 1 teaspoon of mustard and 1 dash of lemon juice)

After that you can also mix everything as you wish ;-)

Shopping list
for 1 week

- [ ] 3 different types of unwashed lettuce
- [ ] 1 package of fresh chicories
- [ ] 4 lbs of tomatoes
- [ ] 1 celery
- [ ] 1 artichoke
- [ ] 5 lemons or 1 bottle of squeezed lemon juice
- [ ] 12 fresh or hard boiled eggs
- [ ] 1 bell peppers
- [ ] 1 cucumber
- [ ] 1 clove of garlic
- [ ] 1 jar of black or green olives
- [ ] 1 can of tuna or anchovies
- [ ] 1 bag of raisins
- [ ] 2 lbs of carrots
- [ ] 2 lbs of apples
- [ ] 1 lb Gruyere or hard cheese
- [ ] 0.2 lb ungrated Parmesan cheese
- [ ] 2 packages of uncut Feta cheese
- [ ] 3 packages of uncut Mozzarella cheese
- [ ] 1 bottle of extra virgin olive oil
- [ ] 1 bottle of balsamic vinegar
- [ ] 1 jar of mustard
- [ ] 1 package of Herb Salt and 1 pepper shaker
- [ ] Basil and oregano
- [ ] Herbs of Provence

Complete tables
to get started...

Here is an example of a completed table:

Date	01.01	02.01	03.01	04.01	05.01
Day	Mon	Tue	Wed	Thu	Fri
Weight*	173.8	173.6	173.4	173.2	173.0
Supper	Caprese Salad	Niçoise Salad	Greek Salad	Caesar Salad	Mixed Salad
Drink	Water	Tea	Juice	Water	Water

Then you'll find enough charts to track the loss of up to 33 lbs!

Date					
Day	Mon	Tue	Wed	Thu	Fri
Weight					
Supper					
Drink					

———————

*Up to 0.1 lb.

Date					
Day	Mon	Tue	Wed	Thu	Fri
Weight					
Supper					
Drink					

Date					
Day	Mon	Tue	Wed	Thu	Fri
Weight					
Supper					
Drink					

Date					
Day	Mon	Tue	Wed	Thu	Fri
Weight					
Supper					
Drink					

Date					
Day	Mon	Tue	Wed	Thu	Fri
Weight					
Supper					
Drink					

Date					
Day	Mon	Tue	Wed	Thu	Fri
Weight					
Supper					
Drink					

Date					
Day	Mon	Tue	Wed	Thu	Fri
Weight					
Supper					
Drink					

Date					
Day	Mon	Tue	Wed	Thu	Fri
Weight					
Supper					
Drink					

Date					
Day	Mon	Tue	Wed	Thu	Fri
Weight					
Supper					
Drink					

Date					
Day	Mon	Tue	Wed	Thu	Fri
Weight					
Supper					
Drink					

Date					
Day	Mon	Tue	Wed	Thu	Fri
Weight					
Supper					
Drink					

Date					
Day	Mon	Tue	Wed	Thu	Fri
Weight					
Supper					
Drink					

Date					
Day	Mon	Tue	Wed	Thu	Fri
Weight					
Supper					
Drink					

Date					
Day	Mon	Tue	Wed	Thu	Fri
Weight					
Supper					
Drink					

Date					
Day	Mon	Tue	Wed	Thu	Fri
Weight					
Supper					
Drink					

Date					
Day	Mon	Tue	Wed	Thu	Fri
Weight					
Supper					
Drink					

Date					
Day	Mon	Tue	Wed	Thu	Fri
Weight					
Supper					
Drink					

Date					
Day	Mon	Tue	Wed	Thu	Fri
Weight					
Supper					
Drink					

Date					
Day	Mon	Tue	Wed	Thu	Fri
Weight					
Supper					
Drink					

Acknowledgements

To my family and my friends
for their precious support.
To Enrique for his precious correction.
To the saleswoman at the Manor in Vevey, in the men's
shirt department, for her precious advice.
To God who makes all things possible.